Scents that Shine

Like the Star:

Celebrity Fragrances for Inspiration

All Natural Perfumery Volume 4

Abigail Houston

ISBN-13: 979-8402546417

ALL BOOKS IN THE ALL NATURAL PERFUMERY SERIES

Scents With Benefits:
How to Craft Fragrances Like a Perfumer, Volume 1

The Essentials of Aroma:
Olfactory, Flavor and Fragrance, Volume 2

You Smell Like a Perfumer:
Creating Natural Fragrances, Volume 3

Scents That Shine Like the Star:
Celebrity Fragrances for Inspiration, Volume 4

Scents at Your Service:
Beneficial Fragrances and Practical Perfumery, Volume 5

High End Scents:
Fine Fragrances and Designer DIY, Volume 6

CONTENTS

CHAPTER ONE
Welcome

Welcome to Volume 4 in the All Natural Perfumery series! Here we venture down the interesting avenues of aroma and apply what we find to blending perfumes. This section along the path of perfumery takes us deep into the woods of an all natural perfumery practice. This book is off the beaten path, the scenic route, the road less traveled, the serendipitous detour, of fragrance creation. This book is a meditation on making a higher connection to our fragrance creations, enlivening our blends with layers of personally significant meaning. Our all natural perfumery hobby totally aligns us with the Law of Attraction — the combination of our favorite smells and concepts, custom curated and prepared with all our best energies — we literally embody the highest vision of ourselves when we wear our special, intentional blend. Our scented personal best, announcing to the Universe, *We Smell Divine.*

I hope this volume isn't too "far out there" for people — we get into frequencies, vibrational aromatherapy, angels, and zodiac signs. We use the words "anoint" and "chakra" a lot here. I looked into each of these different healing modalities in attempts to mine them for relevant information to bring back for perfumery, but be assured I'm not trying to convince you of any belief system, or sell you on some oddball idea. (Other than my books, allow me to sell you on those.)

As I researched the concepts that make up this book, I discovered that each expert has their own ideas about which oils resonate with which chakra/crystal/moon phase/sign of the zodiac, etc. Each author has their own account of how they access the energies of their fragrance materials in ways that are meaningful to them, and what significance they assign to the different healing modalities. Regardless of anyone else's expertise with essential oils or credentials in the healing arts, experiencing and discovering your favorite fragrances is a practice of self discovery. My intention is to inspire your personal perfumery practice as it relates to your individual connection and reflection of mysterious, awesome, eternal Nature.

So please don't get guru vibes coming from me — I'm not trying to claim to have insider metaphysical wisdom or be anybody's spiritual mentor. (Trust me when I say you are really hurtin' for certain if you're looking to me for deep answers on life's great mysteries. Case in point: I'm currently tincturing a Band-Aid.) But I love the fact that people since the beginning of people have been creating fragrances for health and holiness. All natural perfumery increases the magic in your life if you tap into the spiritual.

In this book we get into lots of ways to personalize your fragrance creations so they're really extraordinary, and the best part of volume 4 in the series of All Natural Perfumery is that we get to smell like rich and famous celebrities. Here in perfumery's vortex, we'll harness the awesome power of a Rihanna dupe. Want to elevate your guitar playing? Carlos Santana has a dupe for that. Are your hips accused of lying? Shakira dupe to the rescue. Hungry like a wolf? The Duran Duran dupes say you are in the right place...aligned. Your deepest desire to smell like Gwyneth's hoo-ha? Yes indeedy, right this way. (The Dolly Parton dupe makes no promises though.)

CHAPTER TWO
Let's Review the Basics of All Natural Perfumery

Kendra Grace is an aromatherapist and author who focuses on the psychological and spiritual aspects of perfumery. In her book, *Aromatherapy Pocketbook,* she gives us a quick recap of perfumery's structure. She calls the top notes "flamboyant, bombastic. They make a quick and strong presence. They are important because they add that unforgettable spark to the blend that makes it interesting."

She says the middle notes are used to "round the corners" of your fragrance, "they help equalize oppositions. They are smell mediators, acting as the diplomats of a composition, negotiating chemical balance, and smoothing out differences."

She refers to base notes as, "wise old folks who are calmer, slower, and most times physically denser." She reminds us that base notes help with longevity in all natural perfumery blends.

According to Victoria Edwards, author of *Aromatherapy Companion*, she informs us that the top notes act on the spiritual realm, mid notes have the greatest impact on our emotions, and base notes act on the physical body in spiritual aromatherapy.

Let's do a refresher on the basics of perfumery using Sylvaine-Delacourte as our reference point. She is a perfumer with an outstanding perfumery website. (Her bespoke service is $20k, so she's not just sitting around smelling cute, she means business.) There is tons of info on her blog with links going everywhere, which I've summarized for this perfumery refresher. Her blog is excellent and educational internet quicksand.

"A perfume has an architecture, it is built around an assembly of 5 to 10 components. This is called a chord, just like in music. The main chord gives the theme of the perfume. In a way it is its soul."

Sylvaine-Delacourte's 6 Olfactory Families

Amber — Sylvaine-Delacourte reminds us the classic amber accord is benzoin, cistus labdanum, frankincense, patchouli, sweet myrrh, tonka, and vanilla.

Chypre — says "top and heart notes are rather discreet but then their base notes are intense." Says classic chypre is a "mix of bergamot, jasmine, rose, patchouli, tree moss, labdanum and some animal notes."

Citrus —also called hesperidic.

Ferns Family, commonly called Fougère, which she elaborates is characterized by bergamot, lavender, geranium, rose, oak moss, tonka and vetiver.

Florals — She differentiates green florals (daffodil, narcissus and mimosa), white/sensual florals (high indole jasmine, tuberose, lily, magnolia, orange blossom), spicy flowers (carnation and helichrysum), solar florals (tropicals like ylang ylang, frangipani, tiare), roses (which she includes rose geranium), and powdery florals (example she gives being mimosa).

Woody — "The main natural woody notes are cedar, sandalwood, vetiver, patchouli, pine and cypress." (Abigail here: As a clarifying aside, according to conifer society dot org, the pine family, Pinaceae, is a conifer, thus produces a pine cone. Included in the pine family are fir, spruce, cedars, hemlock and larch.)

Sylvaine-Delacourte explains, "Each main theme, such as woody, floral or citrus, for example, can be dressed in one or more facets. If a perfume is orchestrated with many facets, it is said to be a faceted fragrance. The more faceted it is, the more complex it is, the more surprises it will offer. A not very faceted perfume is more direct and will please more people who seek simple and pure fragrances." She says, "It should be noted that the different accords…can be expressed in a fragrance in the form of olfactory families or in the form of facets," and she goes on to describe olfactive facets in more detail.

Sylvaine-Delacourte's Fragrance Facets

Aldehydic facet — "Enhance freshness and to make the other facets vibrate, especially the floral facet." She describes aldehydic as a more "technical" facet, which I take to mean synthetically engineered. Citrus fruits, especially lime and yuzu are high in aldehydes in all natural perfumery, but the citrus facet and the aldehyde facet are apparently not the same.

Animalic facet — Animal notes were the original fixatives. Beeswax, ambergris (whale intestinal waste), and hyraceum (excrement from a cute African rodent) are the only animal products authorized for perfumery. Herbal musks and "dirty" notes include cumin, costus, cistus labdanum, sage, cedar (atlas), hyssop, and osmanthus.

Aromatic facet — She says aromatic herbs in perfumery add freshness. She elaborates that the 3 subdivisions of aromatic herbs are: lavender notes (which includes hyssop, lavindin, rosemary and thyme), anise notes (which includes anise, tarragon and basil), and minty notes (peppermint, spearmint).

Citrus facet — All citruses fall into this facet, but she highlights bergamot for perfumery, calling it the "fine flower of citrus."

Floral facet — She differentiates six categories in the floral facet.
~Green florals: daffodil, narcissus and mimosa.
~white/sensual florals: high indole flowers— jasmine, tuberose, lily, magnolia, orange blossom.
~spicy flowers: carnation and helichrysum.
~solar florals: tropicals like ylang ylang, frangipani, tiare.
~roses, in which she includes rose geranium.
~powdery florals, the example being mimosa.

Fruity facet — She distinguishes the fruity facet from the citrus facet.
~red fruits: raspberry, strawberry, black currant, blue/blackberries.
~yellow fruits: peach, plum, apricot.
~exotic fruits: coconut, mango, pineapple.
~watery fruits: melons.
~juicy fruits: pear, apple.
She puts fig into an "other fruit" category.
Helpfully, she gives us this blending tip: "Raw materials that are not fruits can still give fruity facets," and she specifies davana, balsam fir, and osmanthus.

Green facet — Vegetal notes. Angelica, galbanum, violet leaf.

Leather facet — Sylvaine-Delacourt's perfumery palette for leather notes: birch, cistus, juniper wood (cade), saffron. She also says everlasting (helichrysum), and cassia cinnamon have leather facets.

Spicy facet —

1. Cold/fresh spices: Cardamom, coriander, juniper berries, pink pepper, ginger (this surprised me, ginger isn't warming?) Cold/fresh spices act more like top notes.
2. Warm spices: Nutmeg, cinnamon wood, black pepper (Piper Nigrum), saffron. The warm spices act more like mid-base notes.

Sylvaine-Delacourte also awesomely informs us that patchouli leaves are odorless until fermented. (I love this kind of info.)

CHAPTER THREE
Modalities for A More Evolved Fragrance

I enjoy learning various methods of healing arts to see how I can integrate their benefits into my life. I read loads of books and online articles written by aroma-energetic practitioners, trying out alternative, vibrational, and esoteric techniques related to perfumery. I learned that the whole point to spiritual perfumery is to make your own connections with your fragrance materials in any ways that feel intuitively meaningful to you. My goal for this chapter is to present healing ideas, systems, and concepts from a wide variety of experts in hopes of inspiring your perfumery creations to greatness.

Let's warm up with a primer on metaphysical basics from Valerie Ann Worwood's book, *The Fragrant Mind* (also annoyingly released as *Aromatherapy for the Soul,* so I ended up buying it twice). Worwood says that when we engage with perfumery on a deeper level, we're practicing what she refers to as 'spiritual blending'. "The good intent of the therapist or person applying the oils activates the light potential in essential oils. Concentrate with love on the plants from which these essences came, on the sacredness of the fragrance, and the joy they bring. These thoughts will be transmitted to the blend." She elaborates, saying essential oils "open the channels of communication, both with the higher self and with higher spiritual elements in the universe."

Energy medicine and healing arts specialist Cyndi Dale educates us that essential oils occupy two states; essential oils are both a liquid and a vapor. Relevant in that aromatherapy connects the limbic system (intuitive/psychic) with the olfactory (sensory) via unique access through the blood brain barrier, elevating perfumery's power to the spiritual realm.

Aromatherapist and author, Candice Covington considers perfumery a form of spiritual alchemy which flows in harmony with established laws of science and nature. One principle of importance in working with essential oils is resonance. Covington notes that humans generate a frequency of 570 trillion times/second (Hz). She explains, "matter is made up of energy vibrating at different frequencies. The human being holds a universe within, filled with overlapping frequencies, and the result is a symphony of cosmic proportions. The principle of resonance describes the way in which one vibration can reinforce another. Resonance builds a vibration that is louder, more stable, or more powerful. When our energetic patterns – our vibrations

– encounter a purer, stronger pattern, the new pattern serves as a template for reformatting the old pattern. A significant key to our well-being and growth is reinforcement of our desired energetic patterns. Essential oils help us achieve the shift in our energetic body that is required for bringing about a deeper, lasting change."

Covington reminds us of The Law of Conservation of Energy, which established that energy can't be created or destroyed, energy can only change form. This law is also called the first law of thermodynamics, and it is how we transfer unhealthy patterns and negative emotions out of our lives, and into powerfully transformative, healing fragrances.

Candice Covington introduces ways to infuse fragrances with vibrational healing energy when resourcing the spiritual side of scent. She encourages perfumers to attend to the subtle energy details of fragrance creation, suggesting we "potentize" our essential oils using "amplification practices." The belief is these practices transmute the healing energies of symbols, sounds, and other ancient concepts, synergistically combining them during preparation, storage, and application of our fragrances.

Numerology

The consciousness of the universe thinks in mathematical codes.
~Kendra Grace

Aromatherapist Candice Covington suggests incorporating the significance of numbers, what she refers to as numerological signatures, when creating fragrance blends. "You can make use of the vibrational energy of numbers in determining the number of drops of an essential oil to use in a blend."

For this next section, I referred to a few tarot books on my shelf that get way into number symbology.

Number 1 symbolizes origin, source, priority, beginning.
Number 2 symbolizes contrast, polarity, divergence, options, partnership.
Number 3 symbolizes triangles, wisdom, teamwork.
Number 4 symbolizes square, solid, structure (there are 4 seasons, 4 directions)
Number 5 symbolizes disorder, chaos, change.
Number 6 symbolizes harmony, order.
Number 7 symbolizes universal truths, challenge, luck.
Number 8 symbolizes strength, boundaries, movement, eternal cycles.
Number 9 symbolizes self mastery, reaching a plateau.
Number 10 symbolizes completion, system reset.

Covington tells us we can further amplify numerological signatures during perfume blending by symbolically using our hands when adding drops of essential oils to invoke either masculine or feminine energy. Covington says adding drops to your blend using your right hand will draw in energetically masculine traits — solar, active, yang, dynamic. Using the left hand while blending your fragrances calls in feminine energies — lunar, receptive, yin, intuition.

Another way we can harness the power of numbers in perfumery is through the golden mean, also referred to as the divine proportion. All throughout nature we appreciate the undeniable beauty of this perfect numerical ratio, reflected as a spiral shape in nautilus shells, snowflakes, and sunflowers. This golden mathematical proportion is the sweet spot of numerical configurations, and we have direct access to it in Fragonia essential oil. As Felicity Warner explains, Fragonia oil is, "remarkable because of its very unusual chemical mix. It's the only oil known to have all of its chemical constituents in almost perfect balance: its oxides, monoterpenes and monoterpenoids form a ratio of 1:1:1," which links "the affinity of Fragonia with cosmic balance and harmony. The golden ratio is an important part of sacred geometry."

Shape Symbols

Covington taps into healing through sacred symbols she calls yantras, which are archetypal shapes, also called the Five Great Elements, or Sacred Geometry. These five sacred shapes represent the eternal ways of nature. The elemental symbols are:

earth — yellow square
water — silver crescent moon
fire — red triangle
air — blue circle
ether/space — black oval

She suggests placing a sticker or other representation of the shape on your fragrance bottle or fragrance storage area/altar to pull in the power of that element to your perfume. Other suggestions for using shape symbols I came up with: draw Reiki symbols on a card, use cards from tarot or oracle decks, take a piece of paper with someone's hand-written signature as a way to infuse their energy into the fragrance, or a piece of favorite artwork.

Planetary Perfumes – Astrology

Perfume shouldn't pollute. Not our bodies or home environments, and certainly not the planet we all share. It appears we'll need something much stronger than all natural perfumery to beat noxious odors on other planets. This Popular Science article title gives us a clue — *What does space smell like? Spoiler: a lot of other planets smell like farts.* Astronauts describe the moon's scent as charcoal, spent gunpowder, and fireplace ashes. "The final frontier smells a lot like a Nascar race — a bouquet of hot metal, diesel fumes and barbecue."

Astrological Perfumes author, James Dotson has curated some guidance for our planetary perfumes. Dotson shares insights about "zodiacal perfumes based on analogies, as well as the archaic and Renaissance correspondences to the seven planets and the four elements."

Earth = heavier scents and base notes.
Air = top notes.
Fire = smokey scents like tobacco and vetiver.
Water = smooth scents (?) and cooling scents. (I think he means like peppermint, spearmint, eucalyptus, wintergreen.)

<u>Aries</u> (planet Mars/element Fire) Warming spices such as pink or black pepper, nutmeg. Coffee. Leather notes. Red flowers (red represents fire).

<u>Taurus</u> (Venus/Earth). Because Aphrodite was born on Cyprus Island, fragrances in the Chypres family correspond. Also palmarosa. Sweet notes like amber, and vanilla.

<u>Gemini</u> (Mercury/Air) Mercury is an androgynous figure, so unisex scents. The gourmand aroma hazelnut belongs to Gemini because "the wand of Mercury was made of hazel nut." Citruses, lavender, mint.

<u>Cancer</u> (Moon/Water) Lunar and night-blooming fragrances like jasmine sambac, ylang ylang and tuberose. Cool, refreshing notes like cucumber, melons, mints. Says myrrh is associated with the moon, so are milky, lactonic notes.

<u>Leo</u> (Sun/Fire) Golden citruses such as orange and mandarin. Warm, sweet spices like cassia and cinnamon.

Virgo (Mercury/Earth) Gourmand notes and pastry accords, because "Virgo holds a sheaf of wheat." Clary sage.

Libra (Venus/Air) Green notes. Geranium. Galbanum.

Scorpio (Mars/Water) Basil, leather notes, pink pepper, sweet myrrh, anise.

Sagittarius (Jupiter/Fire) Jupiter is the "King of Planets," so the "imperial spices" like nutmeg, clove and saffron correspond. Cedar, oak moss. Pear, and peach.

Aquarius (Saturn/Air) Pine and fir. Blue and lavender colored flowers like hyacinth and lavender. "Because it is an electric, scientific and 'modern' sign, all of the aldehydes are Aquarian"(bergamot, lime and yuzu.)

Pisces (Jupiter/Water) Oceanic/aquatic/seaweed. Tropical fruits and flowers like ylang ylang, pineapple, mango.

According to the book *Aromatherapy for Healing the Spirit*, Nicholas Culpeper, the herbalist-astrologer from the 1600's, linked rosemary, frankincense, and laurel (laurus nobilis) to the Sun. He connected jasmine, coriander, and clary sage with the Moon.

Margaret Ann Lembo's book goes into detail about which elements and signs of the zodiac essential oils correspond with, but in her book each zodiac had like 40 oils for each sign, which isn't really helpful. She says that as an Aquarian my protector oil is angelica, and unicorns are my totem animal. She also says that lavender essential oil's totem animals are kittens and puppies. (Her book is filled with this kind of happy hippie talk. I like it, but I don't totally know what to do with it. However, I did learn from Lembo's book that allspice is the universal balancer oil for all of the chakras, so that's something.)

Anointing Rituals

Candice Covington says, "a ritual is a manifestation of intent." For perfumers, these are often referred to as anointing rituals. Anoint is defined as a ritualized blessing, to make sacred. Felicity Warner says to anoint a person is "to dedicate them to serve higher spiritual purpose," and throughout time and culture people have used fragrance anointing rituals to celebrate and elevate the meaningful people and events in life. I've read about bathing rituals and moon phase rituals to enjoy the blessings of daily life. Here are some examples of famous anointing rituals:

Felicity Warner describes the British monarchy's coronation anointing ritual to commemorate the crowning. Warner says the exact recipe is a secret, but describes the coronation oil as rose, jasmine, orange, and cinnamon oils infused in sesame and olive oil carriers.

Celebrity Jennifer Aniston shares her friend circle's anointing ritual: "One tradition I have with my friends is that when one of us gets married, we have a ton of fragrance oils and pretty bottles at the bachelorette party. Everyone puts a drop or two in a bottle for the bride and makes a wish, and the bride wears our creation on her wedding day."

Crystals

A little background about crystals for context: Quartz crystal has physical properties of piezoelectricity, "pressure electricity," the ability to produce electric current/voltage. The phenomena of piezoelectricity occurs when essential oils and quartz crystals are combined. Worwood explains, "piezoelectric effect occurs when pressure is exerted, particularly to crystalline substances, electrical energy is produced. That pressure, or tension can be provided by many things, essential oils are one."

Piezoelectricity is a dependable energy — quartz crystals are used in time keeping, radio transmission, and satellites. As crystal expert Kendra Grace explains, "Thus, information can be carried out in an efficient way without loss of energy."

Aside from the ability to generate electricity, Grace refers to clear quartz as "frozen light" due to its ability to transmit the frequency rates of the entire color spectrum — quartz crystals refract and reorganize light. Grace says clear quartz is the universal healing crystal.

Colors

Grace explains about color frequencies: "All colors each have different rates of vibration and different speeds, or rather, wave lengths. Lower frequencies are the reds and oranges, moving up to the yellows, and higher frequencies are the greens, blues, indigos."

Candice Covington says, "the color spectrum governs different bodies of knowledge," and she explains the following:

*Infrared light governs intuition, which she describes as a "body knowing" and "instinctual perceptions."

*Rainbow colors govern an individual's experiential knowledge, personal karma and causality.

*Ultraviolet light governs archetypal information from Source, the unconscious.

Covington uses different colored bottles to store her oils to enhance her blends with color therapy based on her intentions. If the color blue carries significance for you, blue tansy, blue cypress, German chamomile, and blue yarrow are essential oils that are all vibrant blue in color.

Musical Notes and Sounds

Candice Covington imbues her fragrances with deeper meaning and more powerful intention by chanting sounds called mantras, which are ancient sacred tones. Here are other ways I've gathered to incorporate sound energy while blending or storing fragrance creations to amp up the manifestation energy: reading a poem, playing a song or instrument, reciting an affirmation, ringing a bell, cymbal, gong, or singing bowl.

In 1858, British chemist Septimus Piesse published *The Art of Perfumery,* (Free on Gutenberg.org) where he assigned musical notes to fragrance materials, calling this scale, Octave of Odors. After translating musical notes into fragrance notes, he invented a musical instrument to play them. He called it the odophone or smell organ, and it's described as consisting of "perfume atomizers activated by piano keys, with heavy odors corresponding to low notes, and start odors to the highest notes."

Septimus Piesse's Octave of Odors

B — peppermint, clove, cinnamon
A — lavender, tonka, tolu/Peru balsam
G — magnolia, lilac, orange flower, frangipani
F — ambergris, jonquil, tuberose, benzoin
E — verbena, cedar
D — citronella, bergamot, almond, violet, vanilla
C — pineapple, jasmine, camphor, rose, geranium, sandalwood, patchouli

Candace Pert Ph.D., science researcher and author, assigned musical notes to the chakras. Somehow this will be useful in perfumery.

Chakra	Color	Musical Note
Crown	Violet	B
Third Eye	Indigo	A
Throat	Blue	G
Heart	Green	F
Solar Plexus	Yellow	E
Sacral	Orange	D
Root	Red	C

Chakras

Chakras are the gateways to different levels of our unified field of energy.
~Kendra Grace

Cyndi Dale explains about chakras: "Within and just outside our bodies we have energy centers called chakras. These energy centers process both the psychic (fast), and the sensory (slow) information, feeding this information into our subconscious."

KG Stiles, metaphysician, coach, "Aromatherapist to the Stars," and author of *The Complete Chakra Healing Library,* explains how chakras are wheels of light, sound, and healing. The word Chakra translates from Sanskrit as, spinning wheel of light energy, and Stiles says chakras are, "windows of perception for organizing the various dimensions of reality, and act much like energetic maps or blueprints you use to interpret the meaning of your life experiences."

KG Stiles says these "spiral vortices of energy…your chakras are spinning wheels of energy that connect your physical life form with your transpersonal Divine Nature. Chakras are portals for receiving and perceiving information from the external world. It is at the level of your chakras that you automatically attract, interpret and organize incoming data, as well as transmit vibrational signals and life force energy."

LeAnne Deardeuff, author of *Ultimate Balance: Infusing the Vibrational Energy of Essential Oils into Chakras, Meridians and Organs,* instructs us when working with oils and chakras, you can either apply the essential oils on your hand and wave your hand clockwise above the chakra, or apply your oils directly on your skin where the chakra is located, rubbing your skin clockwise to engage with your chakra energies. (A rollerball or spray application seems easy enough too.)

Chakra and oils expert, Jan Rosenthal, offers this chakra balancing technique: after selecting which oils to interact with, work your way up each of the chakras, "feel where it is 'tight', then gently release the tightness, while calmly considering the things in your life which are causing this tightness."

I consulted a variety of opinions from healing arts professionals so we could get lots of expert input and guidance, but if I just listed all the oils from each author's belief system for each chakra, we'd have about a zillion oils to choose from, and that's not really clarifying or useful. So what I did was, I collated the chakra oil choices from these 3 healing arts experts:

*KG Stiles, "aromatherapist to the stars"

*Kendra Grace, author, aromatherapist

*Valerie Ann Worwood — author of a million books, (*The Fragrant Mind,* also annoyingly released as *Aromatherapy for the Soul,* with different cover artwork even! *So* I was tricked into buying it twice. Not to seem petty, but I want my $20 back. This gnaws my craw enough that I almost didn't use her chakra oil choices, because *Karma*!)

Our 3 experts all perfectly agree on the following exact combos of essential oils + chakra placements. This compilation represents their chakra-oil consensus:

Crown chakra = Frankincense
Brow chakra = Rosemary
Throat chakra = Chamomile
Heart chakra = Bergamot, Ylang Ylang
Solar plexus chakra = Black pepper, Cedar wood, Lemon
Sacral chakra = Lavender, Sandalwood
Root chakra = Myrrh, Patchouli, Vetiver

The oils of neroli, geranium, jasmine, and rose came up a lot among chakra-aroma experts everywhere, not just our 3 experts, however, no one was consistent as to which chakra aligns with which oils. But since Kendra Grace mentioned in one of her books that flowers are heart openers, and since the past five years have been grueling on our heart chakras — what's left of mine is all shriveled — let's add these florals to our chakra fragrance formulation. Our heart chakras totally need hugs.

Additionally, aroma expert Margaret Ann Lembo says allspice is the universal balancer for all the chakras, so into the mix it should go as well. Plus we can't forget to add special, golden ratio Fragonia essential oil to the chakra blend recipe too, since it has such perfectly balanced golden numbers, and will for sure bring us endless miracles upon blessings.

So here's our magical chakra alignment blend using all the oils favored, approved, recommended, and agreed upon by many aromatherapy experts, to keep our chakra wheels happily spinning, all natural perfumery style.

Magical Miracle Chakra Blend

top: bergamot, lemon, neroli
mid floral: chamomile, Fragonia, geranium, jasmine, lavender, rose, ylang ylang
mid herb/spice: allspice, black pepper, rosemary
base: cedar wood, frankincense, myrrh, patchouli, vetiver

Every law of attraction life coach you see online suggests creating a vision board to harness the law of attraction and manifest our dream lives. We can utilize the vision board idea in our perfumery practice by creating a Vision Blend to energize our fragrances with personal meaning and emotion, with the goal of wish manifestation. Amplify our best intentions by adding a crystal, a meaningful object (like a piece of jewelry, scarf, photo), an affirmation, a shape, sound, song, number, color. And with the celebrity scent dupes at the end of this book we can even add our own personal celebrity spokesperson to cheerlead our hippie perfumery crusade.

When we create and wear our specially infused energetic aroma blend, we're projecting our greatest desires into the world, fragrantly announcing our readiness to co-create miracles in our lives. All natural perfumery is a totally interactive, deeply layered engagement with Creation. Your mystical spritz is powerful, and your fragrance creations will sing with clarity and purpose. Amazing, affirming, supernatural magic happens for us when we wear fragrance blends made with this level of care and attention.

CHAPTER FOUR
Complex Fragrance Development

Aromatic compositions mean information
~Kendra Grace, perfumer

Aromatherapy expert Kendra Grace created a therapeutic perfumery method she calls Esscent, "Therapy by aroma," which studies the relationship between memory, emotion and scent. She explains how an Esscent session works:

"I gather the client's smell preferences, the positive associations, in order to blend a custom formulation that serves as a tool in this smell therapy. This perfume contains the best smell associations chosen by the client, going through the different plant parts: roots, resin, wood, leaf, branch, fruit, flower, and seed. The specific aromatic molecules that make up the composition, the personal aromatic signature, feeds into the individual's energy field, transmitting well-being to positively affect body, mind and emotion. This is one of the vibrational healing modalities. Psychotherapy using aroma." By engaging with fragrance in this way, Grace says the perfume creator is composing "a certain harmony having to do with the very best of themselves, then putting that message in a bottle."

In her books she describes the Esscent therapy session process. She guides her clients to smell and rate up to 30 essential oils, notating their preferences on a scale from: -2 for sure rejection, -1 for dislike, 0 for feeling of neutrality, +1 for positive reaction, and +2 for a definite preference. She encourages combining special symbols, sounds, and movements with your scents, and she mentions that an Esscent session also involves crystals and visualizations. Grace considers spiritual perfumery, "your magical act of power."

This next exercise is a modality invented by Valerie Ann Worwood, who specializes in using fragrance for spiritual practice. She developed the "Aroma-Genera Emotional Release" technique, and according to Aroma-Genera practitioner, Pat Antoniak, "It is a system that uses personality types and corresponding essential oils to access physiological or psychological healing and emotional well-being. This system is for expansion, growth."

Here is a summary of Worwood's Aroma-Genera system. Aroma-Genera categorizes people into 9 personality types, sub-grouped into 3 categories:

"Motional Motivators" act before they feel. When emotional they become reactive and action oriented. Their core emotion is anger, and they wish for autonomy. The personality types that belong here are Wood, Root, Resin.

"Emotional Motivators" feel before they act. When emotional they become expressive, dramatic. Their core emotion is guilt, and they wish for attention. Personality types are Herb, Seed, Floral.

"Observational Motivators" They think before they act or feel, and when emotional, they use consideration. Their core emotion is fear, and their core wish is security. Spice, Fruit, Leaf personality types.

Aroma-Genera 9 Personality Types

*Florals want to be admired and have status.

*Fruits want security, respect. She puts citrus, hops, vanilla and tonka here.

*Herbs want appreciation and unconditional love.

*Leaf wants to connect with the environment. Cistus, eucalyptus, patchouli, pine needles.

*Roots are chill and grounded. Ginger, vetiver, turmeric, angelica.

*Resins want position and purpose. Benzoin, Peru/tolu balsams elemi, frankincense, myrrh, copaiba.

*Seeds are creatives, spiritual and intuitive. Star anise, carrot seed, cumin, coriander, nutmeg, fennel, caraway.

*Spices are vivacious and dynamic. Black pepper, cinnamon, clove.

*Woods are loyal and wise, steadfast. Cedar, palo santo, sandalwood.

A note on the Aroma-Genera system is that there's some overlap in categories, examples being lavender is both a floral and herbal, clove is technically the fruit of the plant, cilantro is both a leaf and an herb, coriander is both seed and an herb or spice, etc.

Worwood offers other additional ideas in working with essential oils. For practicing Reiki she suggests two Japanese essential oils, yuzu and hinoki (Japanese cypress). Her book has a section on oils which encourage and support perfumers' communication with angels. In a happy coincidence, all of the Angelic oils on her list also happen to be the oils commonly used in natural perfumery. Angelica oil is the main oil throughout history proclaimed to connect us with angelic guidance, but Worwood also calls on black pepper for protection, carrot seed oil for vision quests, cedar wood for calling in the angels of wisdom, and Roman chamomile for inner peace and joy. (According to her all natural perfumery is a total angel convention).

Worwood shares an exercise on how to experience your fragrance materials: First, waft your scent six inches or so under your nose. Next, emphasize smelling with one nostril, then the other nostril, then both. She says, "When you sniff, inhale the aroma so you can feel it at the very top of your nose." Then Worwood instructs us to visualize the odor traveling through our bodies, following the chain of communication from the essential oil into your nose, through your olfactory system, and along to your brain. Try to perceive the essential oil's effect on your brain's sensory processors and the subsequent healing responses in your physical, emotional, and spiritual bodies. She mystically declares, "The blend performs its own mission."

CHAPTER FIVE
Let's Pick a Perfumer's Nose for Nuggets of Wisdom

This next section goes straight to the source. We thank these professional perfumers for sharing their philosophies on scent and the creative processes that help them express meaning through scent.

Mona Di Orio

Late French perfumer Mona Di Orio (1969-2011) studied architecture and painting, referencing them often during her perfumery career. She was intrigued by the Golden Ratio, the divine proportion, calling it "a key to reach the beauty and the perfect balance. So I have been thinking that it could be fascinating to refer to this theory considering perfume creation." (Me too Late Mona, and I did my best with it a few pages back.)

Her philosophy of fragrance creation is what she calls, "Olfactory Chiaroscuro." Chiaroscuro is the treatment of light and shade in drawing and painting, and as it parallels with perfumery, she explains, "The "lights" are the top notes — the shiny citrus, the sharp green leaves. And with the heart notes we are going to enter slowly in a different mood, to experiment. A different density; more smooth, velvet-like…flowers and spice. And then to reach finally the base notes which are deeper, more intense, sensual, animal and darker."

"I do not like flat perfumes. Some fragrances are linear, they smell the same from beginning to end. It makes me bored, I don't travel, I don't feel a story. I need to feel movement, to follow a development."

Di Orio shared this idea about improving scent awareness when out and about: "The market is the first place I visit when I travel. It informs me about the habits and the customs of the country."

Yosh Han

Yosh Han's website about page describes herself as an aura reading, Reiki practicing, wine sommelier-ing, "super taster" clairvoyant, who is also an award-winning perfumer in San Francisco. In her free time, her bio continues, she participates extensively in water sports. "Yosh made an offering to Poseidon, god of the sea, and committed herself to being an Ambassador of the Ocean."

"I practice vibrational perfumery. Each of my perfumes has an energetic component to them because I design using scent resonance. I don't only focus on the olfactive but also on how the scents work together synergistically, to produce a specific effect spiritually." She teaches her students to, "feel when a fragrance formula is complete. Many people design their formulas from a cerebral place but for me, it's truly about feeling the vibe of a particular scent—if one learns to listen to the raw materials, one can learn to hear the compositions rather than figuring out a mathematical equation. Blending intuitively is very important to me."

Daniel Krasofski

Born in North Dakota, Krasofski says his exposure to Native American culture and the deep connection with nature influences him. He was educated and employed by Aveda, plus many other fancy spa places. According to his LinkedIn profile he is "Currently working with the Hollywood entertainment community to develop scents based on character studies."(I'm pretty sure this means he creates perfumes to help the actors get into character.) "I consider myself a fragrance artist. I explore different ways of engaging our five senses through environment, therapeutic and theatrical scent experiences."

Krasofski likens perfume creation to music. "Utilizing the similarities of music creation to scent creation…when we're creating music we have our top notes, our middle notes and our base notes. And when you put two or more notes together you create an accord. Those accords get put together to create a composition…a full song."

Daniel Krasofski asserts that perfume is similar to wine in that your perfume creation benefits from time to age and mature, and he suggests the perfumer revisit their blend experiments after three months. (*! goodness he's got impulse control*). He also says creating a commercial finished fragrance is a long process—he worked on one project for 1,000 hours. (I blasted out his Aveda dupes in an hour, tops.)

A useful blending tip Krasofski shares is to use frankincense with fragrances where you want to highlight the lemon notes, because frankincense has a lemon facet that will naturally enhance the longevity of top note lemon.

Sabine de Tscharner

Sabine de Tscharner is a scent expert and principal perfumer at Firmenich, the largest privately owned flavor and fragrance company in the world. She advocates for aromatherapy because "fragrances have a proven effect of calming people and bringing them joy."

De Tscharner says market research regarding post pandemic consumer preferences as it relates to the hospitality industry indicates people are looking for clean and comforting scents. Scents considered clean vary by culture, and de Tscharner clarifies, in France lavender is considered a clean scent, but other countries associate lavender with old fashioned fragrances. Tscharner says citrus has global connotations of clean across cultures, and she is excited "to think of new ways to reinvent citrus."

As oranges and lemons are in for a post-pandemic glow-up, she created "what is now her personal favorite fragrance," *Windswept Linen*, marketed to hotels and pubs. Top notes of lemon, sweet orange, and clementine with traces of green ivy*…hints of pine and copaiba wood bring the feel of freshly dried laundry to life…"

*Ivy is described by Fragrantica as "a cool green note with a slightly spicy aspect, very refreshing." Substitute artemisia/davana, spearmint, palmarosa, cardamom, coriander, violet leaf? A clementine is a cross between sweet orange and mandarin/tangerine by the way.

Angelo Orazio Pregoni

This perfumer has done some unusual projects in fragrance creation. In one of his performance art productions he made a perfume out of junk food notes. The article mentioned he used notes like Nutella, fast food burgers, and cola in his junk food fragrance composition, then sold it, not as a finished fragrance, but as a NFT, or some such similarly confusing financial arrangement. (We'll name this fragrance, **Smell Ya Later.**)

Another of Pregoni's unique fragrance projects is his 2013 release of *Peety* perfume, a fragrance that the purchaser personalizes with 1 ml of their own urine. I'm not certain what sort of law of attraction message your "wizz cologne" is supposed to be declaring to the world — something about boundaries and marking territory? A statement of sobriety? Regardless, the notes in *Peety* were listed as: mandarin, jasmine, rose, cinnamon, pink pepper, oak moss, patchouli, sandalwood, tobacco leaf, amber, tonka, your pee.

Sonia Constant

When asked about her methodology for creating a perfume: "First I get inspired by the fragrance's concept, images, words, feeling. Then I imagine some ideas in blocks. They are like planets moving around, like a Calder mobile…"

(Abigail here: *A mobile is a suspended sculpture that utilizes the principle of equilibrium. Calder is an artist who constructed giant mobiles—like each piece is as big as a car, and there are like 10 dangling overhead. Amazing. And then since you're already on google looking up Calder mobiles, check out Calder's Flamingo in Chicago, a stabile sculpture (attached to the ground), as opposed to one of his iconic mobiles (awesomely swaying in the breeze), but a favorite nonetheless. Enough about me fan-girling Calder and gloating about Chicago's incredible wealth of public art. It's back to Sonia…*)

Sonia Constant continues with, "….They are like planets moving around, like a Calder mobile. Some of these blocks meet others, some connect perfectly well together, and some don't. Until there is like a kind of big bang. At that moment, the creative fusion appears and the ideas beautifully merge together. When I look at something inspiring, my brain starts rushing to assemble formulas to create a perfume which would somehow be the echo of what I'm seeing. It is a bit of a synesthetic phenomenon, to appropriate sounds, colors and shapes, and transform them into smell is an incredible chance and infinite source of inspiration."

"If a perfume is well built, you can forget everything surrounding you, the same way you can be subjugated by a landscape, also by looking at a painting or listening to some music. This astonishment can be experienced through perfumes."

"In every artist there lies a scar, a rift, which becomes a source of energy. When you read the biographies of singers and painters and poets and composers, you always notice this rift, this spleen which lent them a poetic sense of life and something beautiful to express. This energy is called resilience. When you're wounded you can either fall, or use the anger and transmute it into something positive."

CHAPTER SIX
Celebrity scents

From what I gather in reading about the celebrity scent industry, the attitude among professional perfumers is that celebrity scents are distasteful, "downmarket," and generally derided as artless money grabs peddled to the lowest common denominator. Celebrity scent PR and marketing expert Kate Morris clarifies, "In most cases the target demographic in the celebrity market is 12-24 year olds. They're young women and girls who will buy the fragrance."

My impression is that most professional perfumers easily and readily accept that a famous celebrity's face will front the ads for designer and house fragrances. But they don't consider a tasteful ad campaign with a classy celebrity from this year's award-winning film nearly the same thing as the fragrance industry offshoot designated as 'Celebrity Scents.'

The conversations surrounding celebrity scents are mostly about how marketing departments are fabricating a 'para-social' relationship between a famous person and the purchasing public through product. Professional perfumers consider the marketing technique of cultivating the illusion of intimacy with a famous person in exchange for perfume sales to young girls, an artistic river too wide to cross. But they often change their tunes, framing it as a "collaboration," because if the celeb isn't too offensive, what kind of fool perfumer would pass up on huge stacks of money and possibly being invited to famous parties?

Perfumer Frank Voelkl says celebrity scents are a "mostly American phenomenon. The fragrance acts as a carrier that connects a consumer to a personality…motivated primarily by obtaining a "piece" of the celebrity and what they represent…and the fragrance has to embody that." Voelkl is "inspired by the spirit of American artists…as they tend to be great pioneers and artistic innovators," specifically naming Norah Jones and Andy Warhol as his personal inspirations. (Frank Voelkl is not a fool perfumer, he created Rihanna's Rogue Man. We do not practice fool perfumery either, we will dupe it).

Chandler Burr, scent critic, creator, and author, says attaching a celebrity to a commercial fragrance saves money for the manufacturer as well as the fragrance house, setting up a lucrative, symbiotic financial relationship. For scale: Richard E. Grant, actor and founder of Jack Perfume said it cost six figures to bring his perfume brand to market. I read Kim Kardashian sold $5 million in 5 minutes with one of her fragrances. Clearly, capitalizing on a celebrity's fanbase can be an enormously profitable business. However, the fragrance market is saturated with an abundance of personality brands attempting to leverage their fame. (Like, who *are* half these people?)

The Celebrity Scents market all started with Parfums Givenchy, founded in 1957, making a splash with the debut of their first fragrance, *L'Interdit*, with ads featuring the great Audrey Hepburn. Perfume historian and blogger Miccaeli says, *L'Interdit* "was the first fragrance with a 'face' — a celebrity who endorsed it in advertising. 'Faces' still exist today for a majority of designer brands, but a celebrity creating their own perfume never succeeded until Elizabeth Taylor."

Miccaeli elaborates on the great Liz T's winning corporate arrangement: "Elizabeth Taylor was the first successful celebrity fragrance franchise. The actress released her first perfume, *Passion* (Elizabeth Taylor, 1987) with the backing of beauty conglomerate Elizabeth Arden. This business model — the celebrity branded perfume line being managed in the shadows by a larger conglomerate — would be the example every celebrity fragrance brand would follow. She famously claimed that her perfumes earned her more than all of her film roles combined. The gold standard had been set."

Two of the earliest fragrances attached to a celebrity that I could find are Brit pop singer Cliff Richard's fragrance, released in conjunction with his 1976 radio hit, *Devil Woman,* and Sophia Loren's Coty fragrance, *Sophia,* which hit the shelves in 1980.

Celebrity scents allow consumers to feel they have insider access to status and fame, however, fragrance expert Nick Gilbert says in a Cosmo interview, "now that has been replaced by social media almost entirely, there is no need to 'buy in' to the lifestyle anymore." In a different interview, perfumer Roja Dove hilariously wondered aloud who is such a fan that they would really want to *smell* like Luciano Pavarotti anyway?

A fragrance expert in a New York Times article kvetches, "Celebrity and big-brand fragrances are too calculated. They use focus groups, and then there are the product managers and PR teams. It gets so far from the celebrity. It's a fake image. Consumers are willing to spend if it's something intellectual."

As hobby all natural perfumers, why would we spend big bank on a dinky bottle of instant migraine? It seems like such a waste of our own perfumery talents, our personal shining stardom of scent. Besides, all your purchase really does is support an ad campaign starring some singer/actress from that disappointing rom-com that dragged on like an hour too long. No thanks, I can sing crappy as I star in my own tedious rom-com. And by the end of this book, using your hobby-level, amateur perfumery skills, you too will be a star, really belting it out through your greatest-hits opening number. Yet you and I will smell fabulously healthy, amazingly natural and powerfully frugal.

Perfumer Geza Schoen, when asked whether celebrity fragrances are vapid, replies: "You can predict the people who are really into fragrances would dwell neither in the juice, nor the idea of a celebrity perfume."

Oh but he would be so wrong about that little prediction. Let us now dwell in both the juices and the ideas of celebrity perfumes.

CHAPTER SEVEN
Formulations

Please enjoy the following celebrity scent recipe templates, listed by date, because we are pop culture historians who also happen to smell famous. Radiate your fragrance dupe like a shining star.

L'Interdit (1957) Givenchy for Audrey Hepburn.
top: bergamot, lime, mandarin, peach, strawberry
mid floral: jasmine, lily-of-the-valley, narcissus, rose, violet, ylang ylang
mid herb/spice: black pepper, clove
base: carrot seed, cistus, frankincense, patchouli, sandalwood, vetiver
sweet: benzoin, tonka

Cliff Richard *Devil Woman* (1976)
top: bergamot, black currant/cassis, grapefruit
mid floral: rose
base: cedar (Virginia), sandalwood
sweet: benzoin, vanilla

Sophia Loren *Sophia* (1980)
top: bergamot, orange
mid floral: jasmine, rose, lang
mid herb/spice: cinnamon, clove
leather notes
base: myrrh, sandalwood, vetiver
sweet: amber, benzoin, vanilla

Catherine Deneuve (1986)
Fifi award winning chypre.
top: aldehydes (lime/yuzu), neroli
mid floral: hyacinth, iris, jasmine, lily valley, rose, violet, ylang ylang
mid herb/spice: galbanum
base: cedar wood (Virginia), musk, oak moss, sandalwood

Cher *Uninhibited* (1987)

top: aldehydes, bergamot, orange
mid floral: geranium, heliotrope, jasmine, rose, ylang ylang
base: cedar, sandalwood, tobacco, vetiver
sweet: vanilla

Mikhail Baryshnikov *Misha* (1989)

top: bergamot, lemon, peach, raspberry
mid floral: carnation, jasmine, rose
mid herb/spice: cinnamon
base: patchouli, vetiver
sweet: amber

Elizabeth Taylor *Passion for Men* (1989)

top: bergamot, lemon, orange
mid floral: carnation, geranium, jasmine, lavender, neroli
mid herb/spice: allspice, anise, cardamom, cinnamon, clove, nutmeg
leather note: fir
base: cedar, oak moss, patchouli, vetiver
sweet: amber, benzoin, tonka, vanilla

Luciano Pavarotti (1994)

top: bergamot, lemon, neroli
mid floral: geranium, rose
mid herb/spice: clove, ivy*, petitgrain
leather: fir
base: cedar (Virginia), frankincense, oak moss, patchouli
sweet: amber, benzoin, tonka, vanilla

Luciano (1999)

top: lemon, orange, tangerine
mid floral: geranium, rose
mid herb/spice: clove, ivy*, lemon verbena, petitgrain
leather: fir
base: cedar (Virginia), myrrh, oak moss, patchouli
sweet: amber, benzoin, tonka, vanilla

The two Luciano Pavarotti fragrance dupes use ivy notes, described as a refreshing, cool, green note. I've used palmarosa, cardamom, spearmint, and coriander as subs.

Andy Warhol *Pour Homme* (1999)

mid floral: jasmine
mid herb/spice: basil, cardamom, tarragon
base: cedar, oak moss, sandalwood

J. Lo *Glow* (2002)

top: grapefruit, orange blossom, neroli
mid floral: jasmine, rose, tuberose
base: carrot seed, copaiba, sandalwood
sweet: amber, vanilla

Heidi Klum (2002)

top: bergamot, mandarin
mid floral: geranium, jasmine
mid herb/spice: nutmeg
base: carrot seed, patchouli, sandalwood, vetiver
sweet: tonka, vanilla

Heidi Klum *Surprise* (2013)

top: mandarin
mid floral: magnolia, rose
mid herb/spice: pink pepper
base: sandalwood
sweet: benzoin

Antonio Banderas *Spirit Men* (2003)
Winner of 2 Fifi Awards in 2005.

top: bergamot, lemon, neroli
mid herb/spice: cinnamon
base: carrot seed, frankincense, patchouli
sweet: amber

Carlos Santana *Men* (2005)

top: apple, bergamot, mandarin, orange
mid floral: lavender
mid herb/spice: cinnamon
leather notes: pines/fir/spruce
base: cedar, cypress, patchouli, sandalwood
sweet: amber, benzoin, tonka

Daisy Fuentes *Dianoche* (2006)

top: lemon, lime, mandarin, orange
mid floral: jasmine, tuberose
mid herb/spice: basil, coriander
base: oak moss
sweet: tonka, vanilla

Paris Hilton *Heir* (2006)

top: bergamot
mid floral: lavender
mid herb/spice: petitgrain
leather: fir
base: patchouli, sandalwood
sweet: amber

David Beckham *Intimately Men* (2006)
Fifi Awards winner 2008.

top: bergamot, grapefruit
mid floral: violet flower
mid herb/spice: cardamom, nutmeg, star anise
base: patchouli, sandalwood
sweet: amber

David Beckham *Beyond* (2015)

top: grapefruit, lime
mid floral: geranium
mid herb/spice: black pepper, cardamom
leather notes
base: cedar, patchouli
sweet: vanilla

Carmen Electra (2007)

top: peach
mid floral: rose
base: cedar, sandalwood

Jenna Jameson *Heartbreaker* (2009)

top: raspberry
mid floral: rose, jasmine, magnolia
base: sandalwood
sweet: amber, tonka

Queen Latifa *Queen* (2009)

cognac
top: bergamot, mandarin
mid floral: jasmine, rose
mid herb/spice: coriander
base: frankincense, patchouli, sandalwood
sweet: tonka

50 Cent *Power* (2009)

mid herb/spice: artemisia/davana, black pepper, coriander, lemon verbena, nutmeg, petitgrain
base: cedar, oak moss, patchouli, sandalwood

Pamela Anderson *Malibu Day* (2009)

top: mandarin
mid floral: honeysuckle
mid herb/spice: pink pepper
base: sandalwood
sweet: amber, caramel, praline, vanilla

Leona Lewis (2009)

top: black currant/cassis, orange, plum
base: cedar (Virginia)
sweet: vanilla

Leona Lewis *Summer Edition* (2011)

top: mandarin, lemon
mid floral: jasmine, rose
base: cedar (Virginia)

Bruce Willis (2010)

top: grapefruit, orange
mid floral: geranium
mid herb/spice: black pepper
base: cedar (Virginia), sandalwood, vetiver

Bruce Willis *Personal Winter Edition* (2016)

top: apple (green), bergamot
mid floral: lavender
mid herb/spice: cardamom, sage
base: cedar, patchouli
sweet: vanilla

Keith Urban (2011)

cognac
top: blackberry
leather: pines/fir/spruce
sweet: amber, chocolate, tonka

Salvador Dali *Fabulous 4* (2011)

top: pear
mid herb/spice: cinnamon
base: frankincense, sandalwood
sweet: amber, vanilla

Salvador Dali *Calice De La Seduction Eternelle* (2015)

top: orange
mid floral: jasmine, rose, ylang ylang
base: cedar, cistus labdanum, patchouli, vetiver
sweet: amber, vanilla

Salvador Dali *Ma Flamme* (2017)

top: bergamot
mid floral: rose
mid herb/spice: artemisia/davana, sage
base: cistus labdanum, sandalwood
sweet: amber

Steve McQueen (2010)

top: apple (green), lemon
mid floral: calendula
mid herb/spice: cardamom, cinnamon, sage
base: cedar (Virginia), patchouli
sweet: amber

Steve McQueen *Legend* (2012)

top: lemon, mandarin
mid floral: geranium, lavender
mid herb/spice: mint
base: cedar, sandalwood, vetiver
sweet: amber, benzoin, tonka

RuPaul *Glamazon* (2013)
mid floral: rose
mid herb/spice: pink pepper
base: cedar
sweet: amber, tonka

Shakira *Wild Elixer* (2013)
top: bergamot, black currant cassis, neroli, peach, tangerine
mid floral: rose
base: cedarwood, patchouli, sandalwood

Jay Z *Gold* (2013)
top: bergamot, blueberry, grapefruit
mid floral: lavender
mid herb/spice: cardamom, ginger, pink pepper, violet leaf
base: myrrh, vetiver
sweet: amber, vanilla

Tim McGraw *Soul2Soul Vintage* (2013)
top: mandarin, orange blossom
mid floral: lavender
mid herb/spice: cardamom, cinnamon, ginger
base: cedar, sandalwood

Rihanna *Nude* (2013)
top: guava, mandarin, pear
mid floral: gardenia, jasmine, orange blossom
base: musk, sandalwood
sweet: vanilla

Rihanna *Rogue Love* (2014)
top: mandarin, peach, red berries
mid floral: honeysuckle, jasmine
base: sandalwood
sweet: amber, caramel, coconut, vanilla

Rihanna *Rogue Man* (2014) Created by Frank Voekl
top: bergamot, clementine
mid floral: jasmine
mid herb/spice: black pepper, rosemary
base: cedar, cistus labdanum, musk, patchouli, sandalwood
sweet: amber, tonka, vanilla

Rihanna *Crush* (2016)
top: bergamot, black currant/cassis, mandarin
mid floral: rose, ylang ylang
mid herb/spice: pink pepper
base: cedar, patchouli

Enrique Iglesias *Adrenaline Night* (2015)
top: lemon, lime, mandarin, plum
mid floral: rose
mid herb/spice: black pepper, cardamom, violet leaf
base: cedar wood, sandalwood, saffron
sweet: tonka

Gwyneth Paltrow's Goop *Edition 01* (2016)
mid: clove
leather: cypress, juniper
base: cistus labdanum, frankincense
sweet: benzoin, vanilla

Gwyneth Paltrow's Goop *This Smells Like My…* (2020)
top: bergamot
mid floral: geranium, rose
base: cedar, ambrette seed* (aka musk mallow).
*I used carrot seed.

Jennifer Aniston *Luxe* (2017)
top: bergamot, tropical sweet berries*, lychee*
mid floral: jasmine, rose
base: carrot seed, patchouli, sandalwood
sweet: tonka
*I subbed in blueberry and guava flavorings.

Dita Von Teese — Heretic *Scandalwood* (2017)
mid floral: rose, ylang
mid herb/spice: carrot seed, cistus labdanum, coriander
base: cedar wood (Atlas), rosewood*, myrrh, sandalwood
*I've recently discovered linaloe wood as a sub for rosewood, but ho wood is great too.

Kim Kardashian KKW *Body* (2018)
top: bergamot, green mandarin, peach
mid floral: jasmine, rose, ylang ylang
mid herb/spice: pink pepper
sandalwood, vetiver, musk
amber

Lionel Ritchie *Hello Men* (2019)
top: bergamot, grapefruit, orange (bitter)
mid floral: lavender
mid herb/spice: mint, violet leaf
base: patchouli, vetiver
sweet: amber

Michael Bolton *Time, Love & Tenderness* (2019)
top: apple (green), bergamot, orange, peach
mid floral: jasmine, rose
base: carrot seed, patchouli
sweet: amber, vanilla

Dolly Parton *Scent From Above* (2021)
top: black currant cassis, mandarin, pear
mid floral: jasmine, lily valley, peony*
leather: fir
base: patchouli, sandalwood
sweet: amber, tonka, vanilla
*Peony is a fantasy floral.

D.S. & Durga collaborations with Duran Duran

Hungry Like the Wolf (2018)
leather notes: pines, juniper (aka cade)
base: atlas cedar, patchouli, sandalwood

Come Undone (2018)
mid floral: rose geranium
base: carrot seed, saffron
sweet: tonka, cacao

A Word About Flankers

The Escentual blog by Thomas defines a flanker as "a fragrance within a franchise — an offshoot of a popular fragrance (a pillar) that brings something new to the series. The purist example of a flanker is a fragrance that takes the olfactory signature of the original and extends it in a natural direction, amplifying key facets and nuances, or subverting them." I read an article in Fragrantica that in 2016, approximately half of all fragrance launches per year were flankers: "fragrances coat-tailing on the success of an established fragrance, retaining part of the name and the packaging design…"

David Beckham

David Beckham's fragrances are strong studies on flankers.

Classic (2013)

top: juniper berry, lime
mid herb/spice: mint, nutmeg
base: cedar (Texas), cypress, galbanum, vetiver
sweet: amber

Classic Blue (2014)

top: apple (green), grapefruit, pineapple
mid floral: clary sage, geranium
mid herb/spice: violet leaf
base: oak moss, patchouli, sandalwood

Aqua Classic (2016)

top: lemon
mid floral: geranium
mid herb/spice: artemisia/davana, cardamom, sage, violet leaf
base: patchouli, vetiver

There are ten flankers in Beckham's *Instinct* series, and six of them are can't-go-wrong super dupes.

Instinct (2005)

top: bergamot, mandarin
mid herb/spice: cardamom, star anise
base: patchouli, vetiver
sweet: amber
*Also called for a spicy habanero pepper note. I omitted this note.

Instinct After Dark (2008)

top: bergamot, grapefruit
mid herb/spice: black pepper, cardamom, petitgrain, star anise
sweet: amber, vanilla

Pure Instinct (2009)

top: citruses, grapefruit
mid floral: lavender
mid herb/spice: black pepper, cardamom, rosemary, sage
base: cedar (Virginia), oak moss, tobacco

Instinct Ice (2010)

top: bergamot
mid floral: geranium
mid herb/spice: black pepper, nutmeg, rosemary
leather: birch
base: elemi, sandalwood
sweet: tonka

Instinct Gold Edition (2015)

top: bergamot, juniper berries, lemon
mid herb/spice: basil, cardamom, rosemary
base: cedar, patchouli, vetiver

Follow Your Instinct (2019)

top: mandarin, orange
mid herb/spice: allspice, cardamom, star anise
base: patchouli, vetiver
sweet: amber

Salvador Dali

Salvador Dali's Le Roy Soleil series does flankers well.

Le Roy Soleil (1998)

top: bergamot, grapefruit
mid floral: geranium, jasmine
base: cedar, rosewood*
sweet: amber
*I used ho wood, and I just discovered linaloe wood, and it's another great sub for rosewood.

Le Roy Soleil Black Sun (2007)

mid floral: clary sage, geranium
mid herb/spice: basil
leather: fir
base: cedar, cistus labdanum, vetiver
sweet: tonka, vanilla

Le Roy Soleil Extreme (2012)

top: apple (green), bergamot, lemon, pineapple
mid floral: lavender
mid herb/spice: cardamom
base: carrot seed, oak moss, vetiver,
sweet: amber

Branded Scents

Landing, United Airline's signature fragrance, diffused in jet bridges, lobbies, lavatories, member lounges, and on hot towels for the fancy first classers. United Airline's "olfactory logo" smells like: bergamot, orange, black pepper, cypress, black tea, sandalwood, and fir.

Virgin Atlantic Airline's signature scent: citrus, rose, eucalyptus and lavender.

Courtney Cox, with fragrance houses Givaudan and Robertet, has launched Homecourt, a line of "fragrance-infused, skincare-inspired, home-care products." Cox claims the signature scent *CeCe*, "is literally the oils that I wear as my perfume," which contains cardamom, cinnamon, "white leather" (substitute with white fir?), mate tea, cedar wood, smoke (maybe sub frankincense or vetiver), and patchouli. Soaps, lotions, surface cleaner, candles, laundry products are retailing from $20 - $50. Her tagline is "Beauty Products for the Home," and I would add, "But Kind of Brutal on My Budget."

Adidas *Urban Spice* (2003) Created by Sabine de Tscharner

top: bergamot, lemon
mid herb/spice: artemisia/davana, cardamom, coriander, mint
leather: birch
base: cypress, patchouli, vetiver

Adidas Sports *STRK For Him* (2019)

top: apple (green), bergamot
mid floral: lavender
leather: birch
base: oak moss, patchouli
sweet: amber, tonka

The Terminator film franchise (2000's)

top: bergamot
mid herb/spice: cardamom, eucalyptus
base: cedar (Virginia), myrrh
*Also calls for a seawater note.

American Idol (2004)
top: bergamot, mandarin, orange
mid: geranium, jasmine, rose, ylang ylang

James Bond (2012) Created by Sonia Constant
top: bergamot, green apple
mid floral: geranium, lavender, rose
mid herb/spice: cardamom
base: oak moss, patchouli, sandalwood, vetiver

Montblanc Emblem (2014) Created by Sonia Constant
top: grapefruit
mid floral: clary sage
mid herb/spice: cardamom, cinnamon, violet leaf
base: sandalwood
sweet: tonka

Grand Budapest Hotel L'Air de Panache (2014)
top: apple (green), bergamot, mandarin
mid floral: jasmine sambac, rose
mid herb/spice: basil, petitgrain
base: carrot seed, cedar, oak moss, patchouli
sweet: amber

Four Seasons London (2012) Created by Roja Dove
top: bergamot, mandarin, orange
mid floral: jasmine, rose
base: vetiver

House of Sillage *Mickey Mouse The Fragrance* (2020)
bergamot, orange blossom, mandarin
mid: cardamom
base: sandalwood
sweet: amber, coconut, cacao, tonka, vanilla

Looney Tunes *Road Runner*
top: bergamot, clementine, guava, peach
base: carrot seed, patchouli
sweet: cacao, tonka, vanilla

Looney Tunes *Wile E. Coyote*

top: bergamot, orange
mid floral: clary sage, lavender
mid herb/spice: coriander
base: carrot seed, cedar, sandalwood
sweet: benzoin, tonka, vanilla

Air/Aroma is a company that specializes in "designing scents for luxury brands," and "translates brand identities into unforgettable signature fragrances." The client brand scent information comes directly from their website, and I list the scent as Air/Aroma has them.

~Barry's Bootcamp workout facilities branded scent smells like: geranium, black pepper, clary sage, eucalyptus, mint, jasmine, rosemary, freesia, cedar wood.

~Ritz Carlton Chicago's branded ambience smells of: rose, green tea, black currant, lemon verbena, "white" jasmine (I take this to mean low indolic, comfortable but not sexy.)

~Swissotel = lavender, cypress, fir, thyme, ylang ylang.

~Dom Perignon = frankincense, cedar wood, patchouli, cistus labdanum, myrrh.

~Hugo Boss in-store scent = bergamot, geranium, basil, coriander, cinnamon, vetiver, oak moss, patchouli, sandalwood.

~Nissan, "first car manufacturer to use scent marketing throughout their automotive trade shows" = bergamot, cardamom, green tea, dry woods.

~Jaguar Land Rover showroom scent = mandarin, orange, rose, Darjeeling tea, cedar wood, leather notes.

Dupes in honor of the professional perfumers we learned from in this book:

Mona di Oria

Eau Absolue (2013)

top: bergamot, mandarin
mid floral: geranium
mid herb/spice: West Indies bay (pimenta racemosa), petitgrain, pink pepper
base: cedar (Virginia), cistus labdanum, vetiver

Vetyver (2011)

top: grapefruit
mid floral: clary sage
mid herb/spice: ginger, nutmeg, patchouli
base: cistus labdanum, vetiver

Vanille (2011)

top: bitter orange
mid floral: ylang ylang
mid herb/spice: clove, petitgrain
mid: leather
base: palo santo, sandalwood, vetiver
sweet: amber, tonka, tolu balsam, vanilla
Called for a rum note so I used vanilla pod rum tincture.

Yosh Han

Sombre Negra (2010)
top: bergamot, lemon
mid herb/spice: artemisia/davana, black pepper, clove, cumin, nutmeg, pink pepper
leather: cypress leaves, juniper
base: carrot seed, cedar wood, frankincense, myrrh, oak moss, patchouli, saffron, sandalwood, tobacco, vetiver
sweet: benzoin, tonka
*Also called for a rum note, so I used vanilla pod rum tincture.

Daniel Krasofski

Aveda Love (1980) jasmine, rose, ylang ylang, sandalwood

Aveda Desert Pure-fume Sand Verbena (2001) citruses, jasmine, ylang ylang, lemon verbena, "green notes"

Aveda Yatra (2007) geranium, lavender, rose, sandalwood

Aveda Pure-fume Pure-formance (2008) lemon, orange, lavender, mint, vetiver

Aveda Chakra Series (2000)

Chakra 1. Motivation—frankincense, patchouli, vetiver

Chakra 2. Attraction—orange, geranium, sandalwood

Chakra 3. Equipose — lavender, fir, lemon

Chakra 4. Fulfillment — mandarin, palmarosa, sandalwood

Chakra 5. Creativity — grapefruit, ylang ylang, rosemary

Chakra 6. Intuition — geranium, petitgrain, orange

Chakra 7. Bliss — angelica, elemi, frankincense

Works Cited

CD Program

Dale, Cyndi. *Energy Clearing,* Sounds True, 2009.

Books

Burr, Chandler. *The Perfect Scent: A Year Inside the Perfume Industry in Paris and New York.* London: Picador, 2009. (This book is follows celebrity Sarah Jessica Parker in developing the scent, Lovely.)

Covington, Candice *Essential Oils in Spiritual Practice: Working with the Chakras, Divine Archetypes, and the Five Great Elements* Healing Arts Press, 2017.

Deardeuff, LeAnne, DC. *Ultimate Balance: Infusing the Vibrational Energy of Essential Oils into Chakras, Meridians and Organs.* Life Science Publishing, 2009.

Edwards, Victoria H. *Aromatherapy Companion.* Storey Books, 1999.

Grace, Kendra. *Aromatherapy Pocketbook.* Llewellyn Publications, 1999.

Grace, Kendra. *Aromatherapy, Crystals & Vibrational Healing.* Nature's Geometry Publications, CA. 2006.

Lembo, Margaret Ann. *The Guide to Aromatherapy and Vibrational Healing.* Llewellyn, 2016.

Lerner, Isha, and Ericksen, Amy. *Tarot of the Four Elements: Tribal Folklore, Earth Mythology, and Human Magic.* Bear & Company, 2004.

Miller, Richard and Iona. *The Magical and Ritual use of Perfumes.* Inner Traditions, 1988.

Mojay, Gabriel. *Aromatherapy for Healing the Spirit.* Henry Holt and Co, 1996.

Pert, Candace, Ph.D. *Everything you need to Know to Feel Go(o)d.* Hay House. 2007.

Piesse, Septimus. *The Art of Perfumery.* (Free on gutenberg.org)

Warner, Felicity. *Sacred Oils: Working with 20 Precious Oils to Heal Spirit and Soul.* Hay House, 2018.

White, Dusty. *The Easiest Way to Learn Tarot Ever.* 2009.

Worwood, Valerie Ann. *Aromatherapy for the Soul* (Also released as *The Fragrant Heavens.* Bad Juju Val.) New World Library, 1999.

Worwood, Valerie Ann. *The Fragrant Mind.* New World Library, 1996.

Websites

Air/Aroma specializes in creating custom fragrances. I took their brand scent client blends from their website.
https://www.air-aroma.com/clients/

Air Esscentuals' blog, "Airline Signature Scent Improves Air In The Air," Virgin Atlantic Airline's signature scent.
https://airesscentials.com/airline-signature-scent-improves-air/

Antoniak, Pat. Natural Comfort Wellness Centre blog, "Aroma-Genera Revisited."
https://naturalcomfort.co/aroma-genera-revisited/

Breaking Travel News, "Bespoke Amenities at Four Seasons Hotel London at Park Lane," 2012.
https://www.breakingtravelnews.com/news/article/bespoke-amenities-at-four-seasons-hotel-london-at-park-lane/

ÇaFleureBon blog, "Frank Voelkl of Firmenich," October 21, 2014.
https://www.ÇaFleureBon.com/interview-with-senior-perfumer-frank-voelkl-of-firmenich-le-labo-santal-33-ylang-49-iris-39-musc-25-baie-rose-26-limette-37-benjoin-19-draw/

ÇaFleureBon blog, "Profiles in American Perfumery: Daniel Krasofski," June 12, 2015.
https://www.ÇaFleureBon.com/ÇaFleureBon-profiles-in-american-perfumery-daniel-krasofski-of-labdk-life-is-an-art-pick-up a brush draw/

ÇaFleureBon blog, "Givenchy L'Interdit," October 6, 2018.
https://www.ÇaFleureBon.com/category/givenchy-linterdit-2018/

Capon, Laura. Cosmopolitan Magazine, "The Death of Celebrity Perfume," Nick Gilbert interview, August 7, 2018.
https://www.cosmopolitan.com/uk/beauty-hair/celebrity-hair-makeup/a22633694/the-death-of-celebrity-perfume-why-no-one-wants-to-smell-like-an-a-lister-anymore/

Chang, Bee-Shyuan. NY Times, "Celebrity Perfumes Get Competition," May 2, 2012.
https://www.nytimes.com/2012/05/03/fashion/perfumers-for-celebrities-start-their-own-lines.html

Dave Lackie website. "Meet Perfumer Sonia Constant," June 14, 2016.
https://davelackie.com/meet-perfumer-sonia-constant/

Dotson, James. "Astrological Perfumes," Sniffapalooza Magazine.
http://www.sniffapaloozamagazine.com/ASTROLOGICALPERFUMESANDVOODOO.html

Fecht, Sarah. Popular Science, "Where Does The Moon's Smell Come From?" August 27, 2014.
https://www.popsci.com/article/technology/where-does-moons-smell-come/

Goller, Richard. "Interview With Perfumer Sonia Constant," Everfumed blog, December 13, 2019.
https://everfumed.com/interview-with-sonia-constant/

H, Alexandre. "The Dreamer — Sonia Constant," The Perfume Chronicles blog, December 19, 2018.
https://www.theperfumechronicles.com/chronicles/soniaconstant

Ilchi, Layla. Courtney Cox Aims to Beautify the Home Category. January 25, 2022.
https://wwd.com/beauty-industry-news/beauty-features/courteney-cox-homecourt-home-brand-details-products-prices-exclusive-1235051093/

Johnson, Dan. "United Introduces New Signature Fragrance," Smart Meetings, March 26, 2015.
https://www.smartmeetings.com/industry_news/united-airlines-introduces-fragrance

Jordan, Julie. *Courtney Cox Launches Her New Home-Care Line Homecourt.* People, January 26, 2022.
https://www.yahoo.com/entertainment/courteney-cox-launches-her-home-140000093.html?guccounter=1

Lane, Heather. "Interview with a Perfumer: A sneak peek 'behind the scents,' LinkedIn, Perfumer Sabine de Tscharner," January 13, 2021. https://www.linkedin.com/pulse/interview-perfumer-sneak-peek-behind-scents-heather-lane/

Lewis, Jessica. "Interview: How Celebrity Fragrances Work," MyDaily UK, May 22, 2015. https://www.huffingtonpost.co.uk/2013/07/18/interview-how-celebrity-fragrances-work_n_7385446.html

Listen to Scents blog, Septimus Piesse info, site now appears defunct.

McGinnis, Chris. "Airlines Take Flight With Branded Scents," SFGate, April 10, 2019. http://msensory.com/airlines-take-flight-with-branded-scents-sfgate/

Miccaeli. "A Cultural Autopsy of the Celebrity Perfume," April 14, 2021. https://miccaeli.substack.com/p/a-cultural-autopsy-of-the-celebrity

NPR, All Things Considered. "Money In A Bottle; The Celebrity Scent Business," Chandler Burr Interview, November 6, 2009. https://www.npr.org/templates/story/story.php?storyId=120183516

Parfumo dot net (for a helpful fragrance notes directory). https://www.parfumo.net/Fragrance_Notes

Perfume Polytechnic, "Thirteen Thoughts — Yosh Han of Yosh Perfumes," December 8, 2015. https://perfumepolytechnic.wordpress.com/2015/12/08/thirteen-thoughts-perfumer-interview-series-yosh-han-of-yosh-perfumes/amp/

Persolaise blog, Richard E. Grant, Jack Perfume, October, 2020. https://persolaise.com/2020/10/richard-e-grant-jack-perfume-live-interview.html

Roche, Pascal. A La Carte Los Angeles, Daniel Krasofski Interview — Ep 9 pt 1, YouTube, July 25, 2016. https://www.youtube.com/watch?app=desktop&v=hGcIqj4vq1Y

Rosenthal, Jan. Garden of Essences blog, chakra balancing exercise. https://gardenofessences.com/articles/chakra-balancing-with-essential-oils/

Schiffman, Lizzie. "What does space smell like? Spoiler: a lot of other planets smell like farts," Popular Science, September 28, 2021. https://www.popsci.com/science/article/2013-07/what-does-space-smell/

Sylvaine-Delacourte company website for a very generous and informational blog. https://www.sylvaine-delacourte.com/en-us/blog?utf8=%E2%9C%93&search%5Bquery%5D=&commit=Search

Symons, Hannah. "Interview Series: Roja Dove, Master Perfumer and Founder of Roja Parfums," Euromonitor Market Research, June 14, 2017. https://www.euromonitor.com/article/interview-series-roja-dove-master-perfumer-and-founder-of-roja-parfums

Thomas, Escentual blog, August 21, 2019. Flankers information. https://www.escentual.com/blog/2019/08/21/5-fragrance-flankers-rival-originals/

Thanks for reading until the end!

Want to increase your perfumery skills and smell even more amazing?

Please come along on another scent adventure with Abigail Houston. In Volume 5, *Scents at Your Service: Beneficial Fragrances and Practical Perfumery*, we apply concepts of perfumery to essential oils typically found in the medicine cabinet. Smell how perfumery turns your apothecary essential oils into artisan fragrance applications. We get all the curative benefits of herbal remedies while smelling like beautiful perfumers.

For more information, visit the website:

AllNaturalPerfumery.com

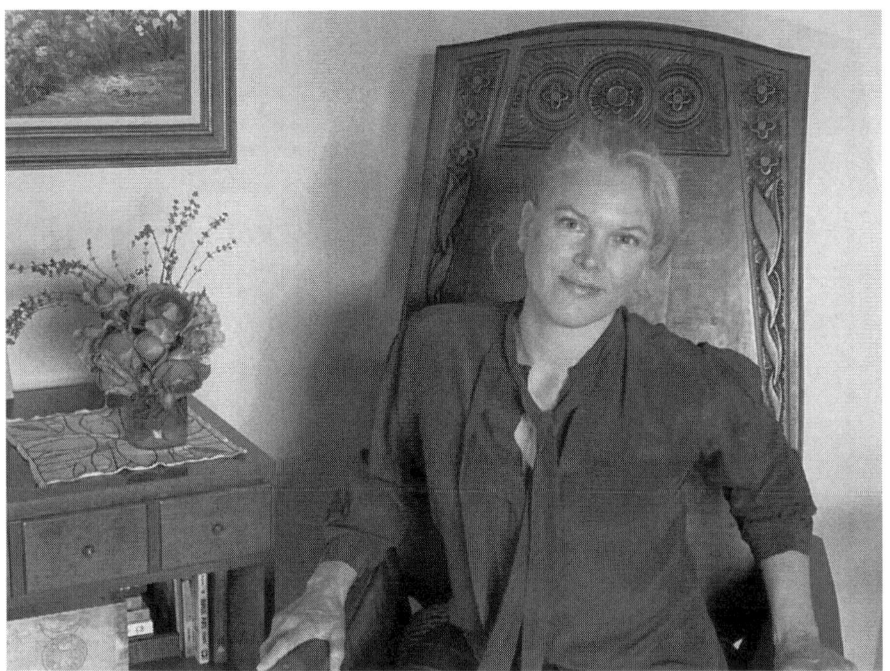

About the Author

Abigail Houston loves personal and home fragrances, but struggles with multiple chemical sensitivities and chronic reactivity. For the past 30 years she's learned and practiced numerous bodywork modalities. Abigail feels that aromatherapy is a timeless healing art and a sustainable solution to environmental pollution. All natural perfumery is her favorite creative strategy to manage the symptoms of modern life. Please join Abigail along the path of perfumery by visiting her website:

AllNaturalPerfumery.com

Made in the USA
Middletown, DE
11 December 2022

18006406R00033